FATTY-LIVER

Fix Delicious Recipes to Support Your Liver

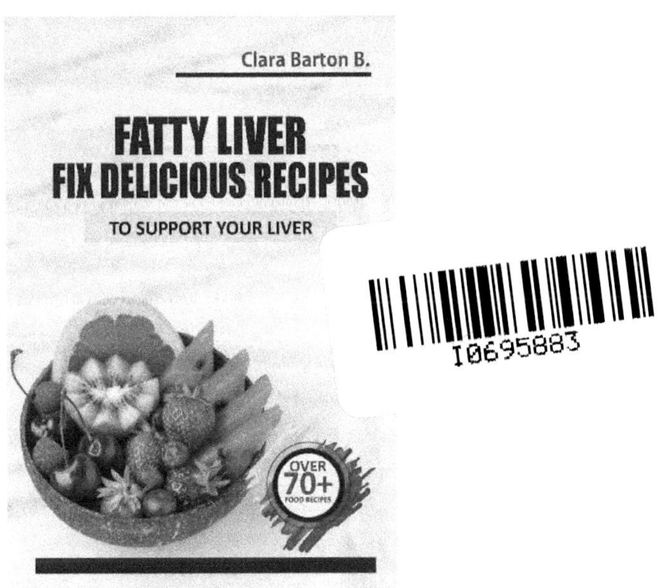

Clara Barton B.

Table of Content

Contents

Introduction

Grasping Fatty Liver Disease

Fatty liver disease, otherwise called hepatic steatosis, is a typical liver condition portrayed by the collection of overabundance fat in liver cells. While some level of fat in the liver is typical, a fatty liver turns into a worry when fat collection surpasses 5-10% of the liver's weight.

There are two principal sorts of fatty liver disease:

1. **Non-Alcoholic Fatty Liver Disease (NAFLD):** This is the most well-known type of fatty liver disease and isn't connected with inordinate liquor utilization. It's frequently connected with metabolic gamble factors like weight, insulin obstruction, type 2 diabetes,

and hypertension. NAFLD can go from straightforward fatty liver (steatosis) to a more extreme condition called non-alcoholic steatohepatitis (NASH), which includes liver irritation and harm.

2. **Alcoholic Fatty Liver Disease (AFLD):** **AFLD** happens because of over the top and delayed liquor utilization. The liver utilizes liquor, and unnecessary admission can prompt fat aggregation in liver cells. AFLD can advance to additional serious liver circumstances, including alcoholic hepatitis and cirrhosis.

Reasons for Fatty Liver Disease:

Metabolic Variables: The most widely recognized reason for fatty liver disease is metabolic condition, portrayed by heftiness, insulin opposition, hypertension, and unusual lipid profiles.

Liquor Utilization: Ongoing and unnecessary liquor utilization can prompt alcoholic fatty liver disease.

Prescriptions: A few meds, for example, corticosteroids and certain disease drugs, can add to fatty liver.

Quick Weight reduction: Fast weight reduction, as found in crash eats less or bariatric medical procedure, can prompt the arrival of fat from fat tissue, which might aggregate in the liver.

Hereditary qualities: Hereditary qualities can assume a part in the improvement of fatty liver disease. A people are more vulnerable because of their hereditary cosmetics.

Side effects of Fatty Liver Disease:

Fatty liver disease is in many cases asymptomatic in its beginning phases. As the condition advances, people might insight:

Fatigue: Stomach distress or torment, particularly in the upper right side

Unexplained weight reduction

Extended liver

Jaundice (yellowing of the skin and eyes) in extreme cases

Fatty liver disease is normally analyzed through a mix of clinical history, actual assessment, blood tests, and imaging concentrates, for example, ultrasound, CT outputs, or X-ray. A liver biopsy might be performed to survey the degree of liver

harm and to recognize NAFLD and NASH.

Treatment and The Executives:

The administration of fatty liver disease principally spins around way of life changes:

Diet: Taking on an eating regimen low in soaked fats, sugars, and handled food varieties while underscoring entire grains, lean proteins, natural products, and vegetables is significant.

Weight The executives: Accomplishing and keeping a solid load through diet and exercise is fundamental, particularly for those with NAFLD.

Standard Activity: Ordinary actual work can assist with further developing insulin awareness, diminish liver fat, and advance in general wellbeing.

Limit Liquor: For people with AFLD, avoiding liquor or diminishing its admission is basic.

Meds: at times, medical services suppliers might recommend prescriptions to oversee explicit parts of fatty liver disease, for example, insulin-sharpening drugs for NAFLD.

Observing: Customary subsequent meet-ups with medical services suppliers and checking liver capability and disease movement are significant.

Fatty liver disease is a typical and possibly serious liver condition. While it vary, may be asymptomatic in its beginning phases, it's fundamental for address risk factors and embrace a liver-accommodating way of life to forestall its movement. Talking with a medical services supplier or an enrolled dietitian is prudent for customized direction and the executives of fatty liver disease.

The Significance of Diet in Liver Wellbeing

The significance of diet in liver wellbeing couldn't possibly be more significant. The liver is a fundamental organ answerable for various basic capabilities in the body, including detoxification, supplement digestion, and the development of proteins vital for blood coagulating. Thusly, what you eat straightforwardly influences the wellbeing and capability of your liver. Here are key reasons featuring the meaning of diet in liver wellbeing:

Upholds Detoxification: The liver assumes a focal part in detoxifying the body by handling and taking out poisons and side-effects. An eating routine wealthy in cell reinforcements and supplements upholds the liver's detoxification processes, assisting it with working ideally.

Controls Fat Digestion: The liver manages the digestion of fats, including the breakdown of dietary fats and the blend of cholesterol and fatty oils. Consuming an eating routine high in immersed fats and refined sugars can prompt fat collection in the liver, adding to fatty liver disease.

Balances Glucose: A decent eating routine manages glucose levels. Unnecessary sugar utilization can prompt insulin opposition and an expanded gamble of creating non-alcoholic fatty liver disease (NAFLD) and type 2 diabetes.

Keeps up with Sound Weight: Keeping a solid load through diet and exercise is vital for liver wellbeing. Heftiness is a huge gamble factor for NAFLD and can prompt irritation and liver harm.

Decreases Irritation: Ongoing aggravation in the liver can prompt liver diseases like hepatitis and NASH. Consuming a mitigating diet wealthy in natural products, vegetables, and entire grains can assist with decreasing liver aggravation.

Advances Supplement Retention: The liver assumes a part in supplement digestion and the combination of proteins required for supplement transport. An even eating routine guarantees the liver has the fundamental supplements to carry out these roles.

Forestalls Liver Disease: A liver-accommodating eating routine can assist with forestalling liver diseases like NAFLD, alcoholic liver disease, and hepatitis. It can likewise sluggish the movement of liver disease in people previously impacted.

Improves Insusceptible Capability: A sound eating routine backings the safe framework, which is fundamental for the liver's guard against diseases and unfamiliar substances.

Decreases the Gamble of Gallstones: An eating routine high in fiber, natural products, and vegetables can assist with forestalling the development of gallstones, which can deter the bile conduits and influence liver capability.

Streamlines By and large Wellbeing: An eating regimen that upholds liver wellbeing frequently lines up with a heart-sound eating routine and general standards of good nourishment. This advances generally prosperity and decreases the gamble of persistent diseases.

In synopsis, a liver-accommodating eating routine is one that is adjusted, wealthy in leafy foods, low in immersed fats and added sugars, and strong of by and large wellbeing. Settling on informed dietary decisions is a proactive method for securing and advance liver wellbeing all through your life. In the event that you have explicit liver worries or conditions, it's prudent to talk with a medical care supplier or enrolled dietitian for customized dietary direction.

Step by step instructions to Utilize This Cookbook

"Utilizing This Cookbook" is a fundamental segment that guides per-users on the best way to capitalize on the recipes and data gave. Here is an example guide on the best way to utilize your Fatty Liver Eating Routine Cookbook:

Instructions to Utilize This Cookbook

Welcome to your Fatty Liver Eating routine Cookbook! This segment will assist you with exploring the cookbook and take full advantage of its recipes and data.

1. Investigate Different Recipes

This cookbook is partitioned into sections that cover different feasts and snacks over the course of the day, including morning meals, snacks, snacks, suppers, sweet treats, and invigorating drinks. Every part contains a determination of recipes intended to take care of various preferences and inclinations. Go ahead and investigate and evaluate new recipes that arouse your curiosity.

2. Follow Nourishing Data

We comprehend that keeping a solid liver is a main concern, and that is the reason we've given nourishing data to every recipe. This incorporates carbohydrate contents, protein content, fiber, solid fats, and carbs. Focusing on these subtleties will assist you with pursuing informed decisions that line up with your dietary necessities and objectives.

3. Adjust to Your Necessities

Now and again, you might have explicit dietary inclinations or limitations, for example, being veggie lover, vegetarian, or having food sensitivities. A large number of our recipes can be changed to accommodate your inclinations. We've included fixing varieties and replacements where appropriate, so make sure to these dishes your own.

4. Dinner Arranging and Part Control

Adjusted and controlled segment sizes are fundamental for keeping a solid liver. Close by every recipe, we've given suggested segment sizes and dietary data. This will assist you with arranging your dinners actually and abstain from indulging.

5. Counsel a Medical care Supplier

In the event that you've been determined to have fatty liver disease or some other ailment, it's fundamental to talk with a medical care supplier or an enrolled dietitian prior to rolling out huge dietary improvements. They can give customized direction in view of your particular wellbeing needs and assist you with coordinating these recipes into your general eating routine.

6. Steady Changes

Addressing your dietary propensities can challenge. Consider rolling out continuous improvements to your dietary patterns. Begin by integrating a couple of liver-accommodating recipes each week and step by step work from that point. Little, reliable advances can prompt enduring enhancements in your liver wellbeing.

7. Keep tabs on Your Development

Think about keeping a food diary to follow your feasts, segments, and any progressions by they way you feel. Observing your dietary decisions and their effect on your wellbeing can be spurring and educational.

Recollect that this cookbook is an asset to assist you with overseeing fatty liver disease and advance generally speaking liver wellbeing. By utilizing these recipes and observing the gave rules, you can make huge strides towards working on your liver wellbeing and by and large prosperity.

GET YOUR COPY...

Blissful cooking, and partake in your excursion to a better liver!

Chapter One: Breakfast Delights

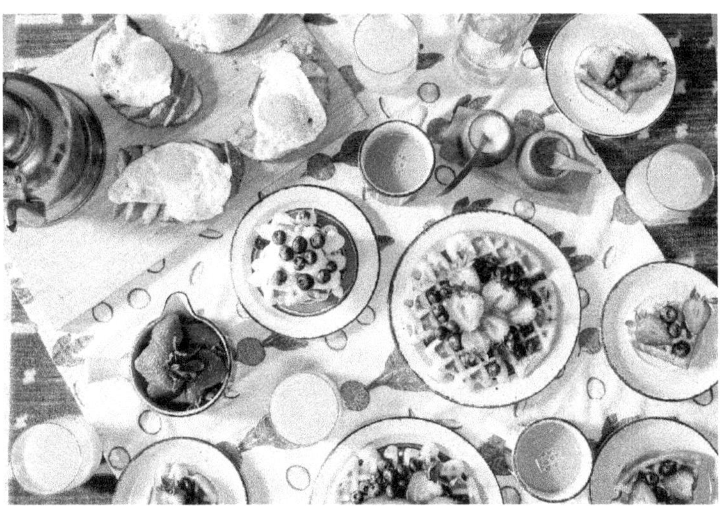

1.1. Oatmeal with Berries

Ingredients:

1/2 cup antiquated oats

1 cup water or milk (dairy or without dairy)

1/2 cup blended berries (strawberries, blueberries, raspberries)

1 tablespoon honey or maple syrup (discretionary)

1/2 teaspoon ground cinnamon

1/4 cup hacked nuts (e.g., almonds or pecans)

A spot of salt

Instructions:

In a pan, heat the water or milk to the point of boiling.

Mix in the oats and lessen the intensity to low. Stew for around 5 minutes, blending every so often, until the oatmeal thickens.

Add a spot of salt and the ground cinnamon. Mix to join.

Eliminate the oatmeal from intensity and move it to a bowl.

Top with blended berries, hacked nuts, and a sprinkle of honey or maple syrup whenever wanted.

Partake in your nutritious and delectable bowl of oatmeal with berries!

Nutritional Combination:

Calories: 300

Protein: 7g

Fiber: 8g

Sound Fats: 6g

Carbs: 54g

1.2   Avocado Toast

Ingredients:

2 cuts of entire grain bread (or your decision of bread)

1 ready avocado

1 little tomato, cut

2-3 radishes, daintily cut

A small bunch of new basil leaves

Salt and pepper to taste

Discretionary garnishes: a sprinkle of red pepper drops, a shower of olive oil, or a press of lemon juice

Instructions:

Toast the cuts of bread until they arrive at your ideal degree of freshness.

While the bread is toasting, cut the avocado down the middle, eliminate the pit, and scoop the tissue into a bowl.

Pound the avocado with a fork and season with a spot of salt and pepper.

When the bread is toasted, spread the squashed avocado equally on each cut.

Top the avocado toast with tomato cuts, radish cuts, and new basil leaves.

Get done with any discretionary fixings you like, for example, red pepper drops, olive oil, or lemon juice.

Serve your lively and delightful avocado toast as a fantastic and nutritious breakfast.

Nutritional Combination:

Calories: 280

Protein: 7g

Fiber: 9g

Solid Fats: 14g

Sugars: 36g

Chapter 2: Wholesome Lunches

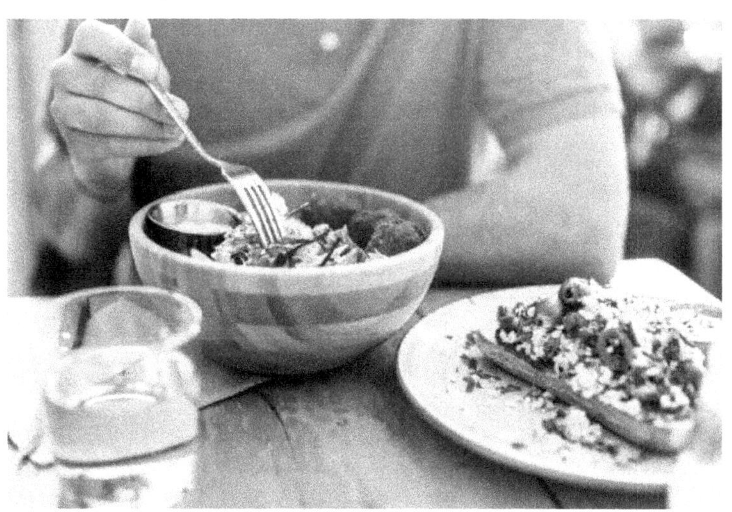

2.1   Grilled Chicken Salad

Ingredients:

2 boneless, skinless chicken breasts

4 cups mixed salad greens (lettuce, spinach, arugula)

1 cup cherry tomatoes, halved

1 cucumber, sliced

1/4 red onion, thinly sliced

1/4 cup chopped fresh basil

2 tablespoons extra-virgin olive oil

1 tablespoon balsamic vinegar

Salt and pepper to taste

Instructions:

Preheat your grill to medium-high heat.

Season the chicken breasts with salt and pepper.

Grill the chicken for 6-8 minutes per side or until the internal temperature reaches 165°F (75°C). Remove from the grill and let it rest for a few minutes before slicing it into thin strips.

In a large salad bowl, combine the mixed greens, cherry tomatoes, cucumber, red onion, and fresh basil.

In a small bowl, whisk together the extra-virgin olive oil and balsamic vinegar to create the dressing.

Drizzle the dressing over the salad and toss gently to coat.

Divide the salad among plates and top with the grilled chicken strips.
Enjoy this delicious and protein-packed grilled chicken salad!

Nutritional Combination:

Calories: 350

Protein: 30g

Fiber: 5g

Healthy Fats: 15g

Carbohydrates: 20g

2.2   Quinoa and Black Bean Bowl

Ingredients:

1 cup quinoa, rinsed and drained

2 cups water or low-sodium vegetable broth

1 can (15 oz) black beans, drained and rinsed

1 red bell pepper, diced

1 cup corn kernels (fresh or frozen)

1/4 cup chopped fresh cilantro

1 teaspoon ground cumin

Juice of 1 lime

Salt and pepper to taste

Optional toppings: avocado slices, Greek yogurt, or salsa

Instructions:

In a medium saucepan, combine the quinoa and water (or vegetable broth). Bring to a boil, then reduce the heat to low, cover, and simmer for about 15 minutes, or until the quinoa is tender and the liquid is absorbed.

In a large bowl, combine the cooked quinoa, black beans, diced red bell pepper, corn kernels, and chopped cilantro.

In a small bowl, whisk together the ground cumin, lime juice, salt, and pepper to create the dressing.

Drizzle the dressing over the quinoa mixture and toss gently to combine.

Serve the quinoa and black bean bowl in individual bowls, and top with optional toppings like avocado slices, a dollop of Greek yogurt, or salsa if desired.

Enjoy this flavorful and nutrient-rich quinoa and black bean bowl!

Nutritional Combination:

Calories: 320

Protein: 12g

Fiber: 10g

Healthy Fats: 5g

Carbohydrates: 58g

Chapter 3: Nutritious Snacks

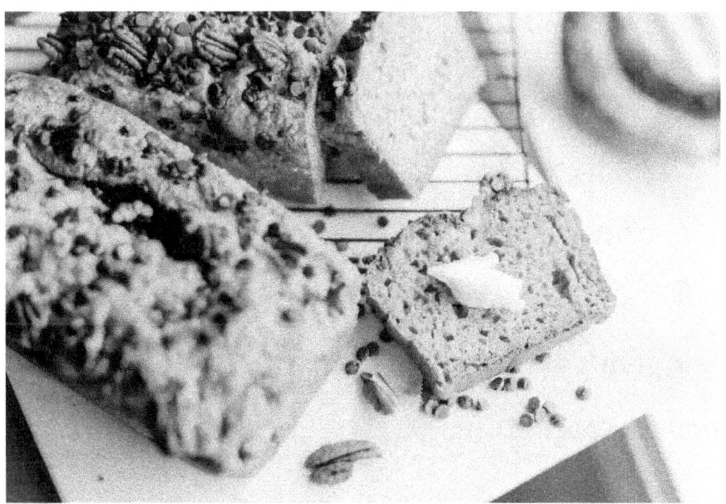

3.1. Greek Yogurt with Nuts

Ingredients:

1 cup Greek yogurt (low-fat or non-fat)

1/4 cup mixed nuts like (almonds, walnuts, and pistachios), chopped

1 tablespoon honey

Instructions:

Spoon the Greek yogurt into a serving bowl.

Sprinkle the chopped mixed nuts over the yogurt.

Drizzle honey over the top for a touch of natural sweetness.

Stir gently to combine, and enjoy this creamy and protein-packed snack.

Nutritional Combination:

Calories: 280

Protein: 12g

Fiber: 2g

Healthy Fats: 18g

Carbohydrates: 20g

3.2. Carrot Sticks with Hummus

Ingredients:

2 large carrots, peeled and cut into sticks

1/2 cup hummus (store-bought or homemade)

Instructions:

Wash, peel, and cut the carrots into sticks.

Serve the carrot sticks with a side of hummus for dipping.

Enjoy this simple, crunchy, and fiber-rich snack.

Nutritional Combination:

Calories: 150

Protein: 4g

Fiber: 6g

Healthy Fats: 7g

Carbohydrates: 18g

3.3. Mixed Berries

Ingredients:

I cup mixed berries (strawberries, blueberries, raspberries)

Instructions:

Rinse the mixed berries under cold water and drain them.

Place the berries in a bowl.

Enjoy this naturally sweet and antioxidant-rich snack as is, or consider adding a dollop of Greek yogurt for extra creaminess.

Nutritional Combination:

Calories: 50

Protein: Ig

Fiber: 5g

Healthy Fats: 0g

Carbohydrates: I2g

Chapter 4: Satisfying Food (Dinners)

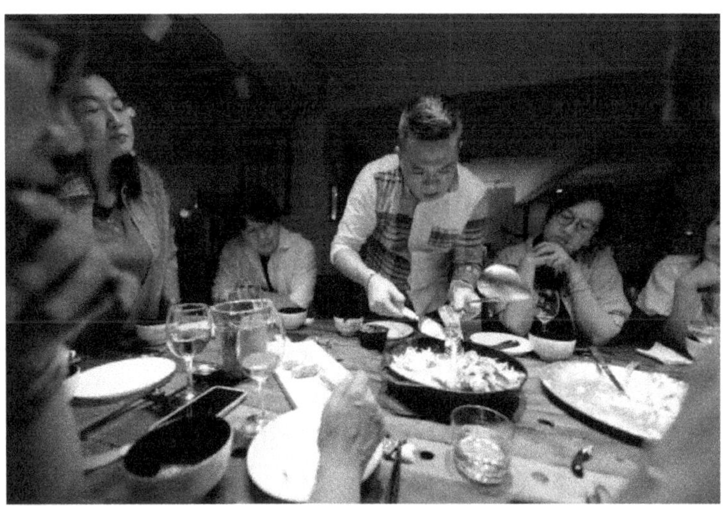

4.1. Baked Salmon with Broccoli

Ingredients:

2 salmon fillets

2 cups broccoli florets

1 lemon, sliced

2 tablespoons olive oil

2 cloves garlic, minced

1 teaspoon dried thyme

Salt and pepper to taste

Instructions:

- *Preheat your oven to 375°F (190°C).

- Place the salmon fillets on a baking sheet lined with parchment paper.

- Arrange the broccoli florets around the salmon.

- Drizzle olive oil over the salmon and broccoli.

- Sprinkle minced garlic and dried thyme over the top. Season with salt and pepper.

- Place lemon slices on top of each salmon fillet.

- Bake for 15-20 minutes or until the salmon flakes easily with a fork and the broccoli is tender.

- Serve hot and enjoy this nutritious and flavorful meal.

Nutritional Combination:

Calories: 350

Protein: 30g

Fiber: 6g

Healthy Fats: 15g

Carbohydrates: 14g

4.2. Stir-Fried Tofu and Vegetables

Ingredients:

1 block extra-firm tofu, cubed

2 cups mixed vegetables (bell peppers, broccoli, snap peas, carrots)

2 tablespoons low-sodium soy sauce

1 tablespoon sesame oil

2 cloves garlic, minced

1 teaspoon ginger, minced

1 tablespoon sesame seeds (for garnish)

Cooked brown rice for serving

Instructions:

+ Press the tofu to remove excess moisture, then cut it into cubes.

+ In a large skillet or wok, heat the sesame oil over medium-high heat.

+ Add minced garlic and ginger and sauté for about 1 minute until fragrant.

+ Add the tofu cubes and stir-fry for 5-7 minutes until they start to turn golden brown.

+ Add the mixed vegetables and continue to stir-fry for another 5 minutes or until the vegetables are tender-crisp.

+ Pour in the low-sodium soy sauce and stir to combine.

+ Serve the stir-fried tofu and vegetables over cooked brown rice, garnished with sesame seeds.

+ Enjoy this delicious and protein-packed vegetarian dinner!

Nutritional Combination:

+ Calories: 380

+ Protein: 18g

+ Fiber: 7g

+ Healthy Fats: 10g

+ Carbohydrates: 48g

4.3. Vegetable and Lentil Soup

Ingredients:

+ 1 cup green or brown lentils, rinsed and drained

+ 4 cups low-sodium vegetable broth

+ 2 cups water

+ 2 carrots, diced

+ 2 celery stalks, diced

+ 1 onion, diced

+ 2 cloves garlic, minced

+ I teaspoon dried thyme

+ I teaspoon ground cumin

+ Salt and pepper to taste

+ Chopped fresh parsley for garnish

Instructions:

+ In a large soup pot, combine the vegetable broth, water, lentils, carrots, celery, onion, garlic, thyme, and cumin.

+ Bring the mixture to a boil, then reduce the heat to low, cover, and simmer for about 25-30 minutes or until the lentils and vegetables are tender.

+ Season the soup with salt and pepper to taste.

+ Serve hot, garnished with chopped fresh parsley.

+ Enjoy this hearty and nutritious vegetable and lentil soup!

Nutritional Combination:

- Calories: 250

- Protein: 15g

- Fiber: 12g

- Healthy Fats: 1g

- Carbohydrates: 48g

Chapter 5: Sweet Treats

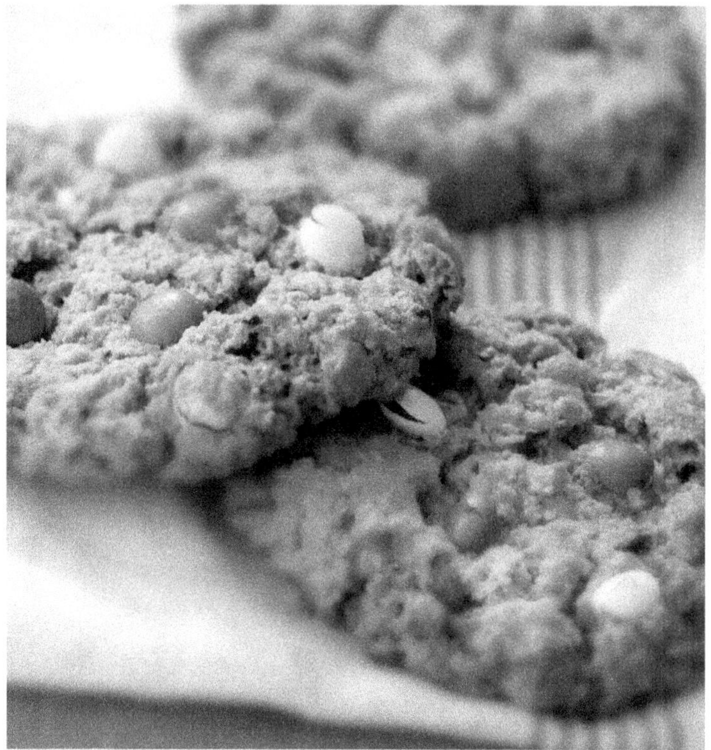

5.1. Baked Apples

Ingredients:

- 4 medium-sized apples

- 1/4 cup chopped walnuts

- 1/4 cup raisins

+ 1 teaspoon ground cinnamon

+ 2 tablespoons honey (optional)

+ 1/4 cup water

Instructions:

+ Preheat your oven to 350°F (175°C).

+ Wash and core the apples, leaving the bottoms intact.

+ In a bowl, combine the chopped walnuts, raisins, and ground cinnamon.

+ Stuff each apple with the walnut and raisin mixture.

+ Place the stuffed apples in a baking dish.

+ Drizzle honey over the top of each apple, if desired.

+ Pour 1/4 cup of water into the bottom of the baking dish.

+ Cover the baking dish with aluminum foil and bake for 30-35 minutes or until the apples are tender.

+ Serve the baked apples warm, and enjoy this naturally sweet and comforting dessert.

Nutritional Combination:

+ Calories: 180

+ Protein: 2g

+ Fiber: 5g

+ Healthy Fats: 6g

+ Carbohydrates: 36g

5.2. Chia Pudding

Ingredients:

+ 3 tablespoons chia seeds

+ 1 cup unsweetened almond milk (or any milk of your choice)

+ 1/2 teaspoon vanilla extract

+ 1 tablespoon maple syrup (or honey)

+ Fresh berries for topping

Instructions:

+ In a bowl, combine the chia seeds, unsweetened almond milk, vanilla extract, and maple syrup (or honey).
+ Stir well to combine all the ingredients thoroughly.
+ Cover the bowl and refrigerate for at least 2 hours or overnight, allowing the chia seeds to absorb the liquid and thicken the pudding.

+ Before serving, give the chia pudding a good stir to ensure a creamy consistency.
+ Top with fresh berries or your favorite fruit.
+ Enjoy this nutritious and naturally sweet chia pudding as a guilt-free dessert or snack.

Nutritional Combination:

Calories: 180

Protein: 5g

Fiber: 10g

Healthy Fats: 9g

Carbohydrates: 21g

Chapter 6: Refreshing Beverages

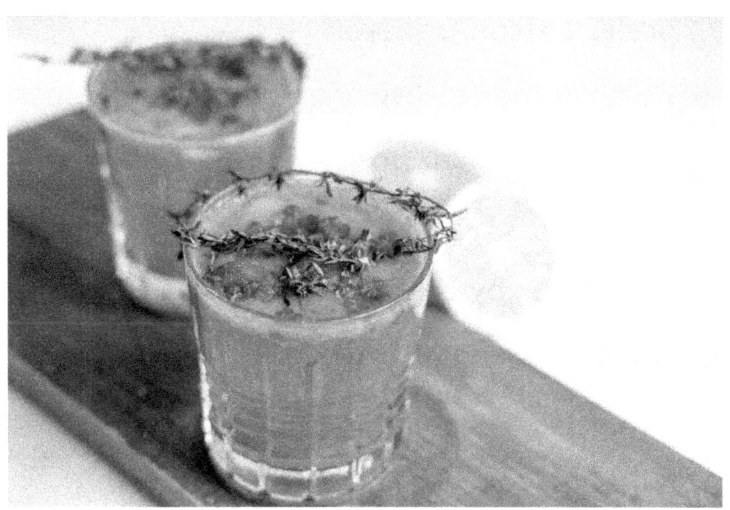

6.1. Green Tea

Ingredients:

+ I green tea bag

+ I cup hot water

Choice: Slices of lemon or a drizzle of honey

Instructions:

+ Place the green tea bag in a cup.

+ Pour hot water over the tea bag.

+ Let it steep for 2-3 minutes, or longer if you prefer a stronger flavor.

+ Remove the tea bag and add slices of lemon or a drizzle of honey for extra flavor if desired.

+ Stir and enjoy this antioxidant-rich, soothing, and liver-friendly beverage.

6.2. Infused Water

Ingredients:

1 lemon, thinly sliced

1 cucumber, thinly sliced

A handful of fresh mint leaves

2 quarts (8 cups) of cold water

Ice cubes

Instructions:

In a large pitcher, combine lemon slices, cucumber slices, and fresh mint leaves.

+ Add ice cubes to the pitcher.

+ Pour cold water into the pitcher and stir gently.

+ Refrigerate for at least 30 minutes to allow the flavors to infuse.

+ Serve this refreshing infused water with ice and enjoy the hydrating and revitalizing benefits.

6.3. Freshly Squeezed Citrus Juices

Ingredients:

+ 2 oranges

+ 2 grapefruits

+ 2 lemons

Instructions:

+ Wash and peel the oranges, grapefruits, and lemons.

+ Cut the fruits into smaller pieces.

+ Use a citrus juicer or a hand juicer to extract the fresh juice from the fruits.

+ Mix the juices in a pitcher.

+ Serve the freshly squeezed citrus juice chilled and enjoy the zesty and vitamin-rich flavors.

Nutritional Combination:

+ Calories: 80 (approx.) per cup

+ Vitamin C: High

+ Antioxidants: High

Conclusion

Keeping a Sound Liver Eating routine

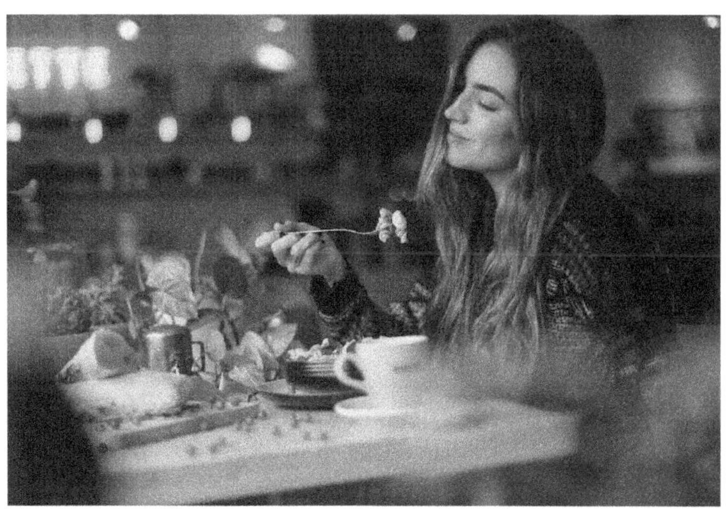

Keeping a sound liver eating routine is critical for supporting liver capability and by and large prosperity. Whether you're hoping to forestall liver disease, deal with a current liver condition, or just advance ideal liver wellbeing, following a liver-accommodating eating regimen is vital. This is an aide en route to keep a solid liver eating regimen:

1. Underline Entire Food sources:

Center around entire, natural food sources like organic products, vegetables, entire grains, lean proteins, and vegetables. These food sources give fundamental supplements and cancer prevention agents that help liver wellbeing.

2. Balance Macronutrients:

Guarantee a fair admission of macronutrients: sugars, proteins, and fats. Pick complex sugars (entire grains) and lean wellsprings of protein (chicken, fish, tofu) while restricting soaked and trans fats.

3. Control Piece Sizes:

Be aware of part sizes to abstain from indulging. Indeed, even quality food varieties can add to weight gain whenever devoured in exorbitant sums.

4. Limit Added Sugars:

Limit the utilization of sweet food varieties and refreshments. Overabundance sugar admission can prompt insulin opposition, a gamble factor for fatty liver disease.

5. Diminish Salt Admission:

Bring down your salt admission to assist with forestalling hypertension and water maintenance. Use spices and flavors for flavor rather than unreasonable salt.

6. Pick Solid Fats:

Remember wellsprings of solid fats for your eating routine, like avocados, nuts, seeds, and olive oil. These fats support liver capability and by and large wellbeing.

7. Hydrate Sufficiently:

Drink a lot of water and hydrating refreshments. Appropriate hydration upholds by and large wellbeing, including liver capability.

8. Limit Liquor Utilization:

Assuming you drink liquor, do as such with some restraint. Unreasonable liquor admission can prompt alcoholic liver disease.

9. Think about Dietary Fiber:

High-fiber food varieties like entire grains, organic products, and vegetables advance solid processing and may assist with decreasing the gamble of gallstones, which can influence liver capability.

10. Cell reinforcement Rich Food sources:

Eat food sources wealthy in cancer prevention agents, for example, berries, citrus organic products, and mixed greens. Cancer prevention agents assist with shielding liver cells from harm brought about by free revolutionaries.

11. Consolidate Liver-Supporting Food varieties:

Incorporate food sources like garlic, turmeric, and artichokes, which have been related with liver medical advantages.

12. Stay away from Handled and Seared Food sources:

Limit the admission of handled food sources, seared food sources, and cheap food. These can add to irritation and liver harm.

13. Counsel an Enrolled Dietitian:

In the event that you have explicit liver worries, it's prudent to talk with an enlisted dietitian who can give customized dietary proposals in light of your wellbeing status and objectives.

14. Continuous Changes:

Rolling out huge dietary improvements can challenge. Consider making steady, reasonable changes to your dietary patterns to guarantee long haul achievement.

15. Normal Active work:

Integrate normal activity into your everyday practice. Active work can assist with overseeing weight, further develop insulin responsiveness, and backing in general liver wellbeing.

16. Screen Progress:

Monitor your dietary decisions and any progressions by the way you feel. Observing your headway can be rousing and assist you with making fundamental changes.